Shedding Pounds:

The Ultimate Straightforward Blueprint To Effortless Weight Loss

By

Eugene C. Allen

Copyright © 2023 by Eugene C. Allen

Table Of Contents

Chapter 5: Having Fun When Working Out

- How important exercise is for weight loss
- How to choose an enjoyable kind of exercise
- Making A Workout Schedule That Matches Your Lifestyle

Chapter 6: Overcoming Obstacles And Maintaining Motivation

- Advice On Getting Over Ruts
- How To Remain Motivated When Losing Weight
- Using Failures As Fuel For Achievement By Learning From Them

Conclusion: Points To Remember

- Finally, Some Inspiring And Motivating Remarks.

Introduction

For as long as she could recall, Emily had trouble with her weight. Everything she had attempted in the way of diets and fitness regimens had failed. Indignant, dejected, and hopeless were her feelings.

She stumbled onto the book "Shedding Pounds: The Ultimate Straightforward Plan to Easy Weight Reduction" one day while browsing social media. She decided to purchase a book since the title piqued her interest.

Emily nodded in agreement with each chapter as she read the book. The author's remarks addressed all the questions and anxieties she had been dragging around for years and spoke directly to her.

She discovered the value of having a positive outlook, developing a sustainable food plan, enjoying exercise, and dealing with setbacks. She was motivated to use the techniques she had learned and to get going.

By making just a few minor dietary and activity modifications, Emily made a tiny start. She concentrated on establishing useful routines and good habits. As a result, she was inspired to keep going since she was finding the process enjoyable.

Emily observed a difference in her physique over many weeks. Even though she had shed a few pounds, she was healthier and stronger than she had been in a long time. She kept moving forward as she continued to heed the recommendations in the book.

Emily marveled at how far she had come months later as she looked back. She had finally lost the weight she had battled for so long, but much more significant was the fact that she had also found her self-worth, learned to love herself and had a fresh outlook on life.

She was appreciative of the advice and encouragement she received from the book "Shedding Pounds" and was aware that it had significantly altered her life.

To help others who are having trouble losing weight, Emily now tells their stories and suggests the book to them. She is aware personally that achieving your objectives and living a better, happier life is attainable.

Why It's Not Always Tough To Lose Weight

Although it might be difficult and time-consuming, losing weight doesn't have to be these things, contrary to popular belief. People often approach weight reduction in an all-or-nothing manner, which is one of the main reasons why they struggle with it.

Many think that to lose weight, they need to entirely change their diet and exercise routine, give up all of their favorite foods, and dedicate hours of their daily schedule to the gym.

The reality is that most individuals cannot maintain this kind of drastic weight reduction. It may be physically and psychologically draining, and long-term maintenance is challenging. A lot of individuals who use this strategy rapidly burn out and go back to their previous behaviors.

Another reason why losing weight doesn't have to be challenging is the fact that even tiny adjustments may have a significant impact. To see results, you don't have to drastically change your food or workout habits. Easy lifestyle adjustments like increasing your water intake, increasing your intake of fruits and vegetables, and taking daily 30-minute walks may make a big difference in your ability to lose weight.

Also, it's crucial to keep in mind that losing weight is about more than simply the number on the scale. It involves altering your lifestyle to improve your general health and well-being.

You'll be more likely to maintain your healthy behaviors over time if you put more effort into developing enjoyable healthy routines than just attempting to lose weight rapidly.

Lastly, while there is no one-size-fits-all method to weight loss, it need not be tough. Since every individual has a unique physique, what works for one person may not work for another.

Choose a weight reduction strategy that suits you by paying attention to your body. Trial and error may be necessary, but the effort will be worthwhile in the end.

In conclusion, weight loss doesn't have to be challenging. You may reach your weight reduction objectives without feeling like you're continuously at war with yourself by adopting a more sustainable and balanced approach to weight loss, making tiny adjustments, and putting an emphasis on overall health and well-being.

The Significance Of Developing A long-term diet and exercise plan

Many individuals make the error of attempting to lose weight rapidly via excessive diets and exercise regimens when it comes to weight reduction.

While this method may provide rapid weight reduction, it is often unsustainable and may have detrimental effects on your physical and emotional health.

Creating a durable weight reduction strategy that is suited to your unique requirements and preferences is crucial for this reason.

A long-term weight reduction program that you can stick to without feeling deprived or overburdened is called a sustainable weight loss strategy.

A sustainable weight-reduction plan's ability to prevent the yo-yo dieting cycle is one of its main advantages. Yo-yo dieting is the practice of rapidly losing weight by drastic methods, only to gain it all back (and sometimes much more) once you resume your routine. This kind of weight loss might harm your metabolism and general health in addition to being annoying.

Your lifestyle and tastes are taken into consideration in a sustainable weight reduction strategy. A strategy that needs you to spend hours on the treadmill each week, for instance, is unlikely to be sustainable if you detest coming to the gym.

Alternatively, a strategy that includes pastimes you like, like dancing, swimming, or hiking, can be more effective. A sustainable weight reduction program focuses on developing healthy behaviors that you can uphold in the long run, which is another advantage.

You are more likely to maintain your food and exercise routines over time if you concentrate on making tiny, incremental improvements to them. Even if you don't lose weight right away as a consequence of this, you may still have improved overall health.

Lastly, a long-term weight reduction strategy is critical for your emotional well-being. It may be emotionally taxing to tackle weight reduction in an extreme way since it can cause emotions of deprivation and restriction.

On the other side, you're more likely to feel good and motivated throughout your weight reduction journey if you develop a sustainable weight loss strategy that incorporates meals you like and activities you love.

In conclusion, the success of long-term weight reduction depends on developing a sustainable weight loss strategy. You may lose weight while maintaining your physical and emotional health by concentrating on small, healthful adjustments that match your lifestyle and interests.

Chapter 1: What You Need to Know About Weight Loss Fundamentals

Understanding the basics of how your body processes food and burns calories might help you lose weight, even if it may seem difficult. You can make better decisions about what you eat and how you exercise and sustainably lose weight by developing a greater awareness of these processes.

Just burning more calories than you eat is the main component of weight reduction. Your body stores extra calories as fat when you eat more than it can burn.

On the other hand, if you expend more calories than you take in, your body will start to use the fat reserves as fuel, which will cause you to lose weight.

Your body's metabolic rate, or how quickly it burns calories, is one of the main elements in weight reduction. Genetics, age, and exercise level are a few of the variables that have an impact on your metabolism.

There are, however, methods to increase your metabolism, such as physical training and consuming meals high in protein.

Understanding how various macronutrients function in your diet is another crucial element of weight reduction. Carbohydrates, lipids, and proteins together make up the three primary nutritional groups known as macronutrients, which provide your body its energy.

Finding the ideal ratio of these nutrients might assist you in achieving your weight reduction objectives since each macronutrient has a unique function in your body.

Your body needs carbs for energy, but not all carbs are made equal. An essential component of a healthy diet is complex carbohydrates, which are found in whole grains, vegetables, and other plant foods.

They give enduring energy. Simple carbs, such as those found in processed meals and sweet snacks, may raise blood sugar levels and should be eaten in moderation.

A balanced diet must include fats, but not all fats are created equal. Unsaturated fats, such as those in avocados and almonds, may decrease cholesterol and lessen the risk of heart disease.

As opposed to unsaturated and trans fats, which may raise cholesterol and increase the risk of heart disease, saturated and trans fats should be ingested in moderation.

Your metabolism may be boosted and weight reduction can be helped by protein, which is necessary for the maintenance and repair of muscle tissue.

In comparison to other protein sources like red meat, lean protein sources like chicken and fish are better for weight reduction since they include fewer calories and saturated fats.

In conclusion, attaining sustained weight reduction objectives depends on having a firm grasp of the foundations of weight loss. You may successfully lose weight in the long run by making educated decisions about what you eat and how you exercise.

This is made possible by knowing about the value of lean muscle mass, the function of macronutrients in your diet, and how to increase your metabolism.

Caloric Intake And Weight Loss

The assessment of the energy your body receives from the food you consume, in terms of calories, is crucial for weight reduction. A calorie deficit, or ingesting fewer calories than your body burns, is necessary for weight loss.

Using a mix of food and activity, one may establish a calorie deficit. The body uses stored fat for energy when you consume fewer calories than it needs to operate, which causes weight loss.

Not all calories are created equal, which is a crucial distinction to make. Although if all calories come from the same source, the kind of food you consume may significantly affect your ability to lose weight.

Fruits, vegetables, and whole grains are examples of foods rich in fiber that may make you feel full and satisfied even when you eat fewer calories. Without feeling hungry or deprived, it may be simpler to achieve a calorie deficit as a result.

Nevertheless, eating a lot of processed carbs or sugar might result in blood sugar spikes, which can trigger cravings and hunger. However, the calorie content of these items may be considerable, which makes calorie deficits more difficult to achieve.

Regarding weight loss, it's also important to pay attention to portion sizes. Overconsumption of even nutritious meals might result in weight gain. You may precisely monitor your calorie intake and make sure you are not overeating by using a food scale or measuring glasses.

Exercise is a vital component in establishing a calorie deficit in addition to nutrition. It is simpler to lose weight if you exercise since it increases metabolism and helps you burn calories. To get the most weight reduction advantages, try to combine cardio and strength training routines.

It's important to keep in mind that having an excessive calorie deficit might be bad for your health. Muscle loss, a slowed metabolism, and dietary shortages may result in rapid weight reduction.

Aim for a modest, consistent weight reduction of 1-2 pounds each week, since this is a healthy and sustainable pace of weight loss.

Finally, it should be noted that calories are quite important for weight reduction. You may shed pounds safely and sustainably by reducing your caloric intake via a mix of diet and activity.

Aim for a modest, consistent weight reduction to reach your objectives while preserving your general health. Pay attention to the sorts of meals you are eating.

The Function Of Metabolism In The Control Of Weight

The word "metabolism" refers to the chemical reactions that take place within the body to maintain its correct operation. Since it controls how many calories your body burns at rest and during exercise, metabolism is important for controlling weight.

Many variables, such as heredity, age, gender, and body composition, have a role in the body's metabolism, which is a complicated process. Although muscle tissue consumes more calories than fat tissue does, individuals with larger muscle mass often have quicker metabolisms.

The idea that metabolism is the only factor in weight growth or reduction is among the most widespread fallacies about it.

The balance between the number of calories ingested and the number of calories burnt via physical activity ultimately determines weight control, even if metabolism does play a part.

Having said that, there are techniques to increase your metabolism to assist your weight reduction objectives. Strength training is one of the best strategies for boosting metabolism.

Your body burns more calories when at rest as a result of strength training's ability to enhance muscle mass. Even when not exercising, this may result in a quicker metabolism and an improved capacity to burn calories.

Consuming certain meals may also help you speed up your metabolism. Lean meats, salmon, and beans are examples of foods rich in protein that need more energy to break down, which temporarily increases metabolism.

By raising body temperature and boosting calorie burn, spicy foods like chili peppers may also aid increase metabolism.

Also, it's crucial to make sure you're getting enough calories to sustain your metabolism. Your metabolism may slow down if you severely limit your caloric intake, which will make weight loss more difficult.

Instead, concentrate on including complete, nutrient-dense foods into your diet and aim for a modest calorie deficit to support your metabolism and general health.

Last but not least, it's important to keep in mind that weight control is a process that demands perseverance and consistency.

A sustainable lifestyle that incorporates good eating practices, frequent exercise, and stress management is the key to long-term success, even if metabolism may play a part.

In conclusion, while it is not the sole element, metabolism is a key component of weight control. You may help your metabolism and reach your weight reduction objectives by including strength exercises, eating meals that speed up your metabolism, and maintaining a modest calorie deficit. To maintain your development over time, keep your attention on developing a sustainable lifestyle.

Foods That Will Support Your Weight Loss Efforts

Your success with weight reduction may be greatly influenced by the kinds of meals you consume. Even though there isn't a miracle meal that will make you lose weight right away, there are several foods that may assist your efforts by improving metabolism, enhancing satiety, and offering vital nutrients to promote overall health.

High-protein foods are one of the finest dietary categories for weight reduction.

While protein is the macronutrient that is believed to be the most satiating, eating less of it might help you feel satiated for longer. Lean meats, chicken, fish, beans, lentils, and tofu are all excellent sources of protein.

High-fiber foods are an additional dietary category that may aid in weight reduction. Fiber is a particular kind of carbohydrate that the body cannot digest, hence it typically makes it through the digestive system undigested.

By making you feel satisfied for longer, you may consume fewer calories overall. Whole grains, fruits, vegetables, nuts, and seeds are all excellent sources of fiber.

Several foods have been shown to increase metabolism and promote weight reduction attempts in addition to those that are rich in protein and fiber.

Among these are hot meals like chili peppers, which include capsaicin, a chemical that may speed up metabolism and enhance calorie burn. Green tea has been demonstrated to enhance calorie burn due to its caffeine and catechin content. Other foods that may speed up metabolism include certain berries, such as raspberries and blueberries, which have anti-inflammatory and weight-loss properties.

Healthy fats should also be a part of your diet since they may help you feel content and full longer, which lowers your risk of overeating. Avocados, almonds, seeds, olive oil, and fatty seafood are excellent sources of good fats.

Instead of depending on processed or high-calorie meals, when it comes to weight reduction, you should concentrate on including full, nutrient-dense foods in your diet.

This may encourage sustained weight reduction while also supporting general health. It's crucial to keep in mind that moderation is the key to successful weight reduction and that no one meal or food type may make or break your efforts.

As a result, increasing your intake of meals that are rich in protein and fiber, foods that speed up your metabolism, and healthy fats may assist your attempts to lose weight. To lose weight sustainably over time, keep in mind to emphasize complete, nutrient-dense meals and to exercise moderately.

Chapter 2: Creating A Solid Base

The secret to success in reaching any objective is laying a solid foundation. This is particularly true when it comes to weight reduction since it calls for modifying one's lifestyle, which may be difficult to maintain without a strong basis.

Numerous crucial elements go into building a solid basis for weight reduction. It is essential to start by establishing definite, defined, and doable objectives. You may use this to stay motivated, give you direction, and keep tabs on your progress toward your final objective.

Building a solid foundation for weight reduction entails not just establishing objectives, but also creating a supportive atmosphere.

In addition to seeking out professional help from a qualified dietician or certified personal trainer, this also entails obtaining social support from friends and family.

During your weight reduction journey, having a support system in place may help you remain accountable and inspired.

Creating healthy behaviors is a crucial part of laying a solid basis for weight reduction.

This includes creating a regular workout schedule, obtaining appropriate rest, and using stress-reduction methods. By lowering stress levels, boosting energy levels, and enhancing general health and well-being, these practices may promote weight reduction attempts.

While building a solid basis for weight reduction, it's equally crucial to concentrate on nutrition. Making nutritious food selections, such as including whole, nutrient-dense foods in your diet and avoiding processed or high-calorie meals is required for this.

To make sure you are remaining within your calorie targets and satisfying your nutritional demands, it may also include measuring your food consumption.

And last, it takes perseverance and patience to create a solid basis for weight reduction. To lose weight, one must often make challenging lifestyle adjustments.

This is not a fast cure. Yet, you may get long-lasting effects and keep a healthy weight over time by concentrating on laying a strong foundation and making durable adjustments over time.

In conclusion, building a solid basis for weight reduction entails establishing specific objectives, cultivating a positive atmosphere, forming wholesome routines, emphasizing nutrition, and exercising patience and tenacity. By following these steps, you may set yourself up for long-term success in your weight reduction endeavor.

Choosing Your Weight-loss Objectives

The first step to a healthier and happier you is to decide what your weight reduction objectives are. Nevertheless, it's not simply a matter of picking a random number off the scale or adhering to the newest diet fad.

Knowing what drives you and what will improve your life can help you develop objectives that are both effective and attainable.

Thinking about why you want to lose weight is the first step in determining your weight reduction objectives. Is it to boost your well-being and lower your chance of developing chronic illnesses like diabetes or heart disease? Is it to boost your self-esteem or to feel more comfortable in your skin? Another reason would be to keep up with your children or grandchildren.

It's time to define concrete, measurable objectives after you have a firm knowledge of your motives. This entails establishing goals that are attainable, practical, and measurable over time.

Instead of stating that you want to "lose weight," for instance, make the objective that you want to "drop 1-2 pounds every week for the next three months."

While establishing weight reduction objectives, it's crucial to take into account your present routines and way of life. Setting a goal to run a marathon may not be the best course of action if you are not already active.

Instead, choose a more manageable, smaller first goal, like walking for 30 minutes each day, three times per week.

It's crucial to define deadlines for completing your objectives in addition to specific ones. This offers a specific goal to strive toward, which encourages responsibility and drive. You could decide to drop 10 pounds, for instance, in the next three months.

Lastly, remember to recognize and appreciate your accomplishments along the road. You may maintain motivation and concentration by breaking down your overall weight reduction goal into smaller, doable objectives. As you reach each goal, celebrate by rewarding yourself with an article of new clothing or just by recognizing your accomplishments.

In conclusion, making clear, quantifiable objectives, taking into account your present habits and lifestyle, creating a timeframe, and enjoying your little victories along the road are all important steps in determining your weight reduction goals. You may position yourself for success and reach your weight reduction objectives by following these steps.

Forming Wholesome Routines And Behaviors

Developing wholesome routines and behaviors is essential for long-term weight reduction success. Making healthy decisions part of your everyday routine helps them develop into habits that are simpler to uphold over time.

Making a plan is the first step in creating healthy routines and behaviors. Create a strategy to integrate the habits you want to develop into your daily routine, such as eating more fruits and vegetables or exercising often.

Starting small is a good strategy for creating healthy habits. Start with one or two bad behaviors you wish to modify rather than your whole lifestyle all at once. If you don't already exercise consistently, for instance, start by committing to a daily brief walk and progressively increase the length and intensity over time.

When it comes to developing healthy routines and habits, consistency is also essential. Strive to incorporate these routines into your everyday life, such as arranging exercises at the same time each day or organizing and preparing nutritious meals for the next week.

Together with creating healthy habits, it's crucial to get rid of bad habits and behaviors that might undermine your weight reduction attempts. This can include consuming less processed meals, staying away from sugary beverages, and consuming less alcohol.

Accountability is a vital component in creating healthy routines and behaviors. Establish a support network, such as a friend or relative who understands your objectives, or sign up for a support group or exercise class. This may keep you inspired and responsible.

Ultimately, it's crucial to have patience and perseverance. It takes time and effort to change routines and habits, and setbacks are common. Don't let tiny failures demotivate you; instead, seize the chance to develop and learn from them.

In conclusion, developing wholesome routines and behaviors is essential for long-term weight reduction success.

Making a plan, beginning small, being consistent, giving up bad habits, finding accountability and support, and being patient and persistent are all necessary to achieve this. By following these steps, you may create wholesome routines and habits that will aid in your attempts to lose weight and enhance your general health and well-being.

Constructing A Support Network

Creating a support network is crucial for anybody hoping to lose weight successfully over the long run. Having a solid support network in place might help you achieve your objectives since losing weight can be difficult.

Finding people you can turn to for help is one of the first stages in creating a support system. This could include close friends, relatives, colleagues, or even a support network. Seek others who are upbeat, supportive, and who share your objectives.

It's crucial to make sure your support system understands your objectives and demands. Inform them of your goals, the kind of assistance you need, and how they can support you in staying on course. This might be seeking assistance with food preparation, exercising, or just offering support and inspiration when you need it the most.

It's important to support oneself in addition to looking for help from others. This might include engaging in self-care tasks like getting adequate sleep, regulating your stress, and carving out time for hobbies you like.

You'll be better able to maintain motivation and concentrate on your weight reduction objectives when you take care of yourself.

Taking a fitness class or enrolling in a weight reduction program is a good approach to developing a support network.

This might provide you access to a built-in network of individuals who support, encourage, and hold you accountable for achieving your objectives. You could also profit from the direction and experience of a qualified coach or teacher.

Furthermore, keep in mind that creating a support network is a continuous effort. Your demands could alter as you go along in your weight reduction journey, and you might need to modify your support network appropriately. Be willing to look for new sources of assistance and modify your strategy as necessary.

Creating a support network is crucial for long-term weight reduction success, to sum up. This entails choosing helpful people, being explicit in your objectives and needs, supporting yourself via self-care, enrolling in a fitness program, and being flexible in changing your strategy as necessary. You can overcome challenges, maintain motivation, and reach your weight reduction objectives with the correct support system in place.

Chapter 3: The Impact Of Attitude

It is impossible to undervalue the influence of thinking on weight reduction. Your thinking will determine whether you succeed or fail in reaching your weight reduction objectives.

Your desire, judgment, and ultimately your capacity to adhere to a weight reduction strategy may all be impacted by your ideas, beliefs, and attitudes toward weight loss.

Positivity is one of the most essential components of thinking. You can remain motivated, make good decisions, and recover from setbacks by adopting a positive mentality.

A pessimistic outlook, on the other hand, might cause emotions of failure, self-doubt, and a lack of desire.

Having a goal-oriented mentality is another crucial component. It's crucial to have realistic, controllable objectives for yourself. Establishing unattainable objectives might result in disappointment and emotions of failure, which can eventually thwart your attempts to lose weight.

It's crucial to concentrate on progress rather than perfection in addition to establishing realistic objectives. Nobody is flawless, and losing weight is a process with its highs and lows.

Remind yourself of your progress and the little successes you've had along the road rather than letting failures demoralize you.

By engaging in mindfulness exercises, you may develop a good perspective. Being mindful requires paying attention to the present and monitoring your thoughts and emotions without passing judgment.

You may learn to recognize negative thinking patterns and swap them out for more constructive ones by engaging in mindfulness practices.

Self-compassion is a crucial component of attitude. Treating yourself nicely and understandingly in the same way that you would a friend will go a long way. Make the most of errors and slip-ups as chances to learn and improve rather than punishing yourself for them.

Finally, keep in mind that changing your mindset is a continuous process. It's a process that goes on forever and needs attention and work.

Continue to create a positive outlook as you go along in your weight reduction journey and look for tools and assistance to keep you on track.

In conclusion, when it comes to losing weight, the influence of thinking cannot be understated. You can remain motivated, make reasonable objectives, keep your attention on your progress, practice mindfulness, have self-compassion, and ultimately succeed in your weight reduction goals by having a positive mentality.

You can change your body and your life by maintaining a positive outlook and being dedicated to your weight reduction quest.

How Your Ideas Might Affect Your Efforts To Lose Weight

Your ability to lose weight may be significantly impacted by your thinking. Your behavior may be influenced by how you feel about food, exercise, and your body, which will ultimately decide whether you are successful or unsuccessful in reaching your weight reduction objectives.

Unhealthy habits, such as emotional eating or missing exercises, may result from negative thoughts like self-doubt or feelings of inadequacy.

Positive attitudes, such as self-assurance and motivation, on the other hand, may motivate healthy behaviors and assist you in sticking with a plan.

Self-talk is one way that your ideas might affect how you lose weight. Your thoughts about yourself have an impact on how you feel and act.

Calling yourself names or making negative comments about your appearance may lead to emotions of guilt and poor self-esteem, which can sap your drive and make it more difficult to maintain good behavior.

On the other side, constructive self-talk may increase self-esteem and support constructive conduct.

Cognitive distortions are another way that your ideas might influence your efforts to lose weight. Negative thought processes known as cognitive distortions may result in illogical thinking and undesirable actions.

All-or-nothing thinking, catastrophizing, and black-and-white thinking are a few examples of cognitive distortions. For instance, "I can't have any sweets ever," or "If I eat this doughnut, I'll gain 10 pounds," are examples of all-or-nothing thinking.

Negative thinking patterns of this kind might make it difficult to maintain healthy routines and promote emotional eating or bingeing.

Lastly, by affecting your expectations, your ideas might influence your weight reduction journey. You may be setting yourself up for disappointment and frustration if you have unreasonable expectations regarding weight reduction, such as expecting to lose a lot of weight soon or wanting your body to appear a specific way.

Unhealthy habits like severe dieting or over-exercising might result from unrealistic expectations.

Self-awareness and mindfulness practices are crucial for developing a good mentality and overcoming negative thinking habits. Pay close attention to how your ideas and feelings affect you.

Negative ideas should be contested and replaced with optimistic ones. Consider progress rather than perfection. Furthermore, keep in mind to be kind and understanding toward oneself.

In conclusion, your ideas might significantly affect your efforts to lose weight. Positive ideas may motivate healthy actions and assist you in reaching your weight reduction objectives, whilst negative thoughts can cause unhealthy behaviors and make it more difficult to maintain good habits. You may change your ideas and your body to succeed long-term in your weight reduction journey by exercising self-awareness, confronting negative thinking patterns, and developing a positive mentality.

Guidelines For Cultivating An Optimistic Outlook

Success in all areas of life, including weight reduction, depends on cultivating a positive outlook. Thoughts of negativity and self-doubt are simple to fall prey to, but by using a few straightforward techniques, you can teach your mind to concentrate on the positive and develop a more upbeat view.

Here are some ideas for cultivating a good outlook when trying to lose weight:

Engage In Acts Of Gratitude: Gratitude is a powerful technique for refocusing your attention from what you lack to what you do have. Spend some time every day thinking about the blessings in your life, whether it's a kind friend or family member, a cozy house, or your resiliency and fortitude.

Create Attainable Objectives: Achieving attainable goals is essential to boosting confidence and preventing discouragement. Instead of attempting to implement a significant change all at once, set tiny, attainable objectives that build upon one another. During the process, be proud of your progress, no matter how modest it may appear.

Visualizing success is a useful strategy for boosting confidence and drive. Spend some time each day picturing yourself reaching your weight reduction objectives, whether that means looking and feeling better in your favorite pair of pants or just being more at ease in your skin. You are more inclined to take action to make it happen if you can see success more often.

A positive company can do wonders for your outlook, so try to surround yourself with positive people. Avoid negative or criticizing friends and family members and seek out those who are encouraging and helpful.

Joining an online forum or support group for weight reduction may also be a terrific way to meet others who share your interests and are working toward the same objectives.

No one is flawless, including you, so keep your attention on development rather than perfection.

Instead of aiming for perfection, concentrate on development. No matter how little they may appear, acknowledge your accomplishments, and draw lessons from your failures. Keep in mind that failures are a natural part of any journey and do not determine your success.

Practice Self-care: Developing a positive mindset requires that you take good care of your physical, mental, and emotional needs. Make time to engage in enjoyable hobbies like reading, listening to music, or having a soothing bath. Prioritize getting adequate sleep and eating nutritious meals, and practicing stress-relieving exercises like yoga or meditation.

Negative thoughts are a normal part of the human experience, but that doesn't mean you have to believe them. Instead, you should challenge them.

Challenge negative thoughts by asking yourself if they are true or if there is confirmation to support them. Then, replace negative thoughts with positive affirmations that reinforce your self-worth and confidence.

By incorporating these tips into your daily routine, you can develop a more positive mindset that will support you in achieving your weight loss goals.

Remember that cultivating a positive mindset takes time and effort, but with persistence and dedication, you can transform your mindset and achieve success in all areas of your life.

Strategies For Overcoming Common Mental Roadblocks

When it comes to losing weight, the biggest roadblocks are often mental. Negative thoughts, self-doubt, and fear of failure can all stand in the way of achieving success.

Fortunately, there are several strategies you can use to overcome these mental roadblocks and stay on track with your weight loss goals.

Determine Your Triggers: Knowing your triggers is one of the first stages to overcoming mental obstacles. What circumstances or feelings make you more likely to slide downward? Knowing your triggers can help you create tactics to avoid them.

Practice Mindfulness: Being completely present and aware at the moment is the practice of mindfulness. It may assist you in maintaining your attention and preventing the distraction of unfavorable or self-doubting thoughts.

Consider adding mindfulness practices like meditation or deep breathing into your everyday routine.

Negative ideas may be reframed because although they are a normal part of the human experience, they don't have to dictate how you behave. Try turning negative remarks into ones that are more productive and positive.

Reframe your thoughts, for instance, to "I'm capable of making good changes and attaining my objectives" rather than "I'll never be able to lose weight."

Appreciate Minor Victories: Recognizing your progress may keep you inspired and committed to your objectives. It's important to recognize even little successes, like increasing your water intake or going for a 10-minute stroll. No matter how little it may appear, progress is progress.

Create A Network Of Support: When it comes to conquering mental obstacles, having a support network of friends and family members may be helpful. Consider joining a weight loss support group or online community, as well as reaching out to loved ones for encouragement and support.

Create Reasonable Expectations: The key to preventing disappointment and annoyance is to create reasonable expectations. Remind yourself that losing weight is a slow process and that setbacks are common along the way. Consider progress rather than perfection, and acknowledge each incremental success as it occurs.

Visualizing achievement might help you overcome obstacles in your mind and maintain motivation.

Spend some time each day picturing yourself reaching your weight reduction objectives, whether that means looking and feeling better in your favorite pair of pants or just being more at ease in your skin. You are more inclined to take action to make it happen if you can see success more often.

By combining these techniques into your weight reduction journey, you may get beyond frequent mental obstacles and continue moving in the direction of your objectives. Keep in mind that losing weight is a process, so be patient and nice to yourself as you go. You can succeed despite any mental obstacles if you are persistent and committed.

Chapter 4: Planning A Sustainable Meal

One of the most crucial elements in attaining long-term weight reduction success is developing a sustainable food plan. With the aid of a meal plan, you may make better food decisions, meet your calorie targets, and resist the need to eat on the spur of the moment.

You may develop a sustainable meal plan that will assist you in achieving your weight reduction objectives and maintaining a healthy lifestyle with a little forethought and preparation.

Establishing your calorie requirements is the first step in developing a sustainable food plan. Depending on your age, gender, weight, and degree of exercise, this will change. You may determine your daily calorie demands with the aid of many online calculators.

Foods that are abundant in nutrients and low in calories are referred to as nutrient-dense foods. Fruits, vegetables, lean meats, whole grains, and healthy fats are included in this.

Your body will get the nutrients it needs to operate correctly while you feel fuller for a longer period thanks to these meals.

You may remain on track with your calorie targets and prevent impulsive food choices by planning your meals. Spend some time every week organizing your meals and snacks for the next week.

Batch cooking is a fantastic method to save time and make eating healthily more practical. Choose a day of the week to prepare many meals ahead of time, then store them in the refrigerator or freezer for later in the week.

Don't Overlook Snacks: Eating healthy snacks helps keep you full between meals and prevent overeating. Choose protein- and fiber-rich snacks like Greek yogurt with berries or carrot sticks with hummus.

Be Adaptable: Having a food plan is crucial, but so is being adaptable. There may be moments when you need to modify your strategy because life occurs. Be ready to adapt as necessary, and don't be hard on yourself if things don't go exactly as you had planned.

Get Expert Advice: If you're having trouble coming up with a sustainable food plan, think about getting advice from a licensed dietitian or nutritionist. They can assist you in coming up with a customized food plan that suits your particular requirements and tastes.

For sustained weight reduction, developing a sustainable food plan is crucial. You may design a meal plan that matches your lifestyle and aids in the achievement of your objectives by selecting nutrient-dense foods, organizing your meals in advance, and being adaptable.

While you work towards being a healthier, happier version of yourself, keep in mind to be patient and nice to yourself along the road. Furthermore, remember to enjoy each tiny triumph.

Having An Awareness Of Portion Size

To lose weight healthily, it's essential to comprehend portion management. On our calorie intake and rate of weight loss, the size of the food portions we eat may have a big influence.

A calorie deficit may result in malnutrition and other health issues whereas an excessive calorie intake, even from nutritious meals, can cause weight gain.

Understanding how much food your body needs to function properly is essential for portion management. It may be difficult to do this in a culture that often favors consuming excessively big portions of food.

You may create healthy habits and achieve your weight reduction objectives, however, by learning to manage your portions.

This advice will assist you in comprehending portion control:

Use Visual Signals: One of the simplest methods to manage your portions is by using visual cues. A portion of pasta, for instance, should be the size of a tennis ball, but a dish of meat should be comparable to a deck of cards. While cooking or eating out, use these visual clues to gauge portion sizes.

Study the nutrition facts on food labels to learn about portion sizes. They often include details about serving sizes and calorie counts. While you buy groceries and prepare meals, pay attention to these labels.

Using smaller dishes might help you eat fewer calories, according to research. Instead of feeling the urge to overfill a bigger plate, utilizing a smaller plate may help you feel more satiated with fewer quantities of food.

Eat Mindfully: Mindful eating means being aware of your hunger signals, eating gently, and relishing your meals.

You may better manage quantities and prevent overeating by being more conscious of your eating behaviors.

Be Prepared: You may manage your portions by planning. Choose a healthy alternative that is within your calorie objectives from the menu before you go out to dine. Use measuring spoons and cups while cooking at home to make sure you're putting out the right amount of food.

Depriving yourself of the meals you like may often backfire and result in overeating. Let yourself indulge in little amounts of your preferred meals instead.

You won't feel as deprived and are more likely to adhere to your healthy eating plan if you allow yourself to enjoy your favorite foods in moderation.

Finally, for long-term weight reduction, it's essential to comprehend portion management. You may form healthy habits that will help you manage your portions and achieve your weight reduction goals by utilizing visual cues, reading food labels, using smaller plates, practicing mindful eating, making plans ahead of time, and refraining from deprivation.

Always keep in mind that portion management is all about finding a balance that suits your body and your lifestyle, so be patient and gentle to yourself as you work toward your objectives.

Guidelines For Meal Planning And Preparation

Anybody wanting to make better decisions and maintain their nutrition goals will find meal planning and preparation to be a very beneficial tool. When you're pressed for time or unprepared, it may help you save money, avoid making poor food choices, and save time.

Understanding your goals is one of the most crucial components of meal planning and preparation. Together with any particular dietary preferences or limits you may have, this also covers your general health objectives.

A list of the nutritious items you like to eat should be made when you have a clear knowledge of your objectives and an inventory of your kitchen.

Your meal plan will be built around this, and by including foods you like, you'll be more likely to stick with them.

Portion management is a key component of meal preparation. You may prevent overeating and make sure you're getting the right quantity of nutrients for your body's requirements by knowing how much food constitutes a good portion.

To do this, you may use measuring cups, a food scale, or even just your mind's eye to picture the right amount of food.

There are many tactics you may use to simplify and streamline the meal preparation process. Uncomplicated grab-and-go choices throughout the week may be easily achieved by cooking bigger quantities of meals and storing them in separate containers.

Another useful strategy is to schedule meal preparation on a specified day and prepare your menu in advance.

A comprehensive nutrition plan should include both meal preparation and planning for your snacks. Snacks might help you feel fuller and less prone to overeating during meals.

Choose protein- and fiber-rich snacks, such as a piece of fresh fruit, some hummus-topped vegetables, or a handful of almonds.

Meal planning and preparation may, in general, be a very effective technique for helping you lose weight. You may make a sustainable meal plan that will aid in your long-term success by being aware of your objectives, exercising portion control, and using smart tactics.

Dietary Guidelines And Recipes For Effective Weight Reduction

Making food choices might be one of the most difficult aspects of starting a weight reduction plan. Fortunately, there are many nutritious and delectable meal suggestions and recipes that may support your weight reduction efforts.

Emphasizing full, nutrient-dense foods like fruits, vegetables, whole grains, and lean meats is one well-liked strategy for a balanced diet. Salads, stir-fries, and bowls are just a few of the meal options that may help you do this.

For individuals wishing to consume more vegetables, salads are a fantastic alternative. Use kale, spinach, or arugula as a substitute for the traditional greens, and include a range of vibrant vegetables like carrots, peppers, and cucumbers.

Add a lean protein like grilled chicken or tofu on top, along with a nutritious dressing prepared with olive oil, lemon juice, and herbs.

Stir fries are another quick and delectable supper option that may be tailored to your preferences. Broccoli, snow peas, and mushrooms make a good vegetable basis. Next, add a protein, such as tofu or shrimp.

Garlic, ginger, and soy sauce may be used for taste when cooking with healthy cooking oil, such as avocado oil.

The meal option of a bowl may be customized to your liking and is flexible and filling. Toppings like roasted veggies, black beans, and avocado may be added to a foundation of quinoa or brown rice.

Add some tahini or yogurt-based healthy sauce on top, along with grilled chicken or fish or another lean protein.

You can also find a ton of nutritious recipes online that can aid in your weight reduction efforts in addition to these meal suggestions.

Don't be scared to use your imagination in the kitchen while experimenting with new tastes and ingredients.

Your overall nutrition objectives and dietary limitations should be taken into account when choosing recipes or meal suggestions.

Consider speaking with a trained dietitian if you want more help. Strive for balanced meals that contain a range of dietary categories.

Weight reduction may be a pleasant and joyful process with the appropriate recipes and meal plans. You may reach your weight reduction objectives and boost your general health and wellness by concentrating on full, nutrient-dense meals and experimenting with new tastes and ingredients.

Chapter 5: Having Fun When Working Out

Many individuals see exercise as a necessary evil that must be completed to reduce weight or maintain their health. Yet it isn't always the case. In truth, if you approach exercise correctly, it may bring you joy and satisfaction in life.

Choose things that you like and look forward to performing if you want to enjoy exercising. From yoga to dance to hiking, this can be done.

You'll be more likely to continue with them and incorporate fitness into your daily life if you choose pleasurable hobbies.

Making exercise a communal activity is one strategy for enjoying it. Attend a group exercise class or look for a workout partner who has similar interests.

Exercise with a friend or group may keep you motivated, provide you support and accountability, and just generally be more fun.

Focusing on your feelings while exercising rather than simply your physical outcomes is another approach to enjoying it.

Exercise causes the production of endorphins, which improve mood and lessen tension and anxiety. You may develop a more fulfilling and long-lasting connection with the exercise by paying more attention to how it makes you feel than merely the number on the scale.

It's also critical to approach exercise with a development perspective as opposed to a fixed one. Exercise should be seen as a chance to push yourself, acquire new abilities, and advance personally rather than as something you must do to attain a certain result.

This might alter your viewpoint and make working out more pleasurable and fulfilling.

Making exercise a sustainable part of your life is crucial, too. To do this, you must strike a balance between pushing yourself and taking care of your body.

Pay attention to what your body requires and change your exercises appropriately. Always keep in mind that exercise is just one part of a healthy lifestyle.

Your physical, mental, and emotional health may all be enhanced by finding enjoyment in exercising. You may have a lifelong, fulfilling relationship with exercise by doing things you love, making it a social activity, concentrating on the feelings it gives you, adopting a development mentality, and making it a sustainable part of your life.

How important exercise is for weight loss

While it's not simply about burning calories, movement is crucial for weight reduction. The advantages of activity extend well beyond the purely physical, and they may aid you in making permanent progress toward your weight reduction goals.

First and foremost, exercise and physical activity are crucial for enhancing general health and lowering the risk of chronic illnesses including cancer, diabetes, and heart disease.

Together with other advantages, regular exercise helps strengthen your heart, lungs, and immune system.

But, exercise especially is important for weight reduction. You burn calories when you move your body, which may help you reduce your caloric intake and lose weight.

Yet, exercise has advantages that extend beyond calorie burning. Regular exercise may also help you burn more calories, raise your metabolism, develop more muscle, and improve your body composition, all of which can result in long-term weight reduction.

The importance of movement for lasting weight reduction may also have a significant influence on one's mental and emotional health. Endorphins are released when you exercise, and they may lift your mood and lessen tension and anxiety.

Frequent exercise has also been associated with enhanced cognitive function, better sleep, and higher levels of self-assurance and self-esteem.

Movement is vital for weight reduction since it helps establish healthy routines and habits in addition to the physical and psychological advantages.

Making exercise a regular part of your day increases your likelihood of making other healthy decisions, such as selecting wholesome meals and getting enough sleep, throughout the day.

The ability to change your thinking and connection with your body is possibly the most significant reason why exercise is essential for weight reduction.

You may develop a healthy and long-lasting connection with movement and with yourself by moving your body in ways that feel pleasant and helpful instead of punitive or restricting. Long-term motivation and dedication to your weight reduction objectives might be supported by this.

Moreover, it should be noted that although the activity is important for weight reduction, it doesn't merely include calorie burning.

You may lose weight in a healthy, sustainable way while simultaneously enhancing your general health and wellness thanks to the many physical, mental, and emotional advantages of exercise.

Making exercise a regular part of your life can help you develop healthy habits, speed up your metabolism, enhance your body composition, and develop a good and long-lasting connection with your body and movement.

How to choose an enjoyable kind of exercise

Exercise is an important component of weight reduction and will aid you in reaching your objectives. However, a lot of individuals find it difficult to find an exercise they love, which makes them less motivated and inconsistent with their regimen. Choose hobbies that you like and that make you feel good since this is why it's so important.

Many possibilities exist for physical exercise, ranging from conventional gym workouts to extracurricular activities and outdoor sports. Find what function for you by experimenting.

Maybe you like to exercise in a communal setting with Zumba or yoga, or maybe you prefer more solitary pursuits like cycling or jogging.

The fact that exercise doesn't have to be a chore must also be kept in mind. You may look forward to it every day as an enjoyable and sociable activity. Think about signing up for a team in a sport, enrolling in a dancing class, or even simply taking a buddy on a stroll.

Setting attainable objectives and establishing a reliable habit is just as crucial as discovering pleasurable hobbies. Set modest objectives at first, such as taking a daily stroll or once a week trying a new fitness class, and then gradually increase the duration and frequency over time. For exercise to become a habit and to provide lasting effects, consistency is essential.

Do not misjudge the value of rest and recuperation. For your body to heal and regenerate, injury prevention strategies such as stretching and rest days are essential. Physical activity may become a sustainable and fun component of your weight reduction journey by selecting a workout you love and developing a regular regimen.

Making A Workout Schedule That Matches Your Lifestyle

To reach your weight reduction objectives, you must develop an exercise program that works with your lifestyle. Finding a regimen that works for you while taking into consideration your tastes, limits, and schedule is key.

Think about your timetable and everyday activities first. What time of day are you most attentive? Do you follow a set routine or a flexible schedule? While preparing your fitness schedule, keep these things in mind.

Make an effort to plan your exercises during the morning hours if you have more energy. If your workday is hectic, try to squeeze in quick exercises during your breaks or after you finish.

Consider what kind of exercise you both like and can accomplish physically next. Low-impact exercises like swimming or cycling may be beneficial for you if you have joint discomfort or mobility issues.

But if you like intense exercises like HIIT or CrossFit, include them in your program. It's crucial to choose activities that you love, is challenging for you, and are good for your body.

Setting attainable objectives and progressively increasing your exercise volume and intensity over time is also crucial. If you aren't used to it, don't attempt to start a demanding fitness regimen.

Begin with a couple of days each week and add more until you have a more regular schedule. To avoid becoming bored and to keep your body challenged, you might vary your routines.

Remember to take relaxation and recuperation into account, too. Schedule rest days, including stretching and foam rolling in your regimen, and give your body time to recover from exercises so it can heal and regenerate.

You may make physical activity a lasting and pleasurable component of your weight reduction journey by designing an exercise program that suits your tastes and way of life. Finding a balance that works for you and advances your objectives rather than pushing yourself to the edge every day is the key.

Chapter 6: Overcoming Obstacles And Maintaining Motivation

It's not always simple to lose weight. Despite your best efforts, it's possible to encounter obstacles that might make you feel demotivated and disappointed. These setbacks may take many different forms, such as emotional eating, a weight reduction plateau, or a lack of energy or ambition to work out.

While setbacks are a normal part of any weight reduction journey, it's crucial to keep in mind that you can overcome them and maintain your motivation. The secret is to address setbacks with the appropriate mindset and tactics.

Reassessing your objectives and reminding yourself of why you began your weight reduction journey in the first place is an excellent method.

Are you hoping to become healthier, look better in an article of certain clothing, or feel better about your appearance? Whatever your motivation, it's critical to keep it front of mind to keep you moving forward.

Celebrating your accomplishments, no matter how tiny they may appear, is another useful tactic.

Did you complete a difficult workout? Were you manage to resist the urge to indulge in a sweet treat? Enjoy these little victories and utilize them to gain momentum toward your ultimate objective.

A solid support system should be in place as well. Be in the company of individuals who will encourage and motivate you when you need it and who will be supportive of your efforts to lose weight.

Think about signing up for a support group or hiring a personal trainer who can provide direction and responsibility.

It's also critical to understand and control your triggers. Does emotional eating or a lack of drive to exercise tend to be brought on by any particular circumstances or emotions? Make a strategy to handle these triggers after identifying them.

Ultimately, it's important to cultivate self-compassion and kindness toward oneself. Always keep in mind that setbacks are a common part of any weight reduction journey, and it is OK to take a pause or change your objectives as necessary.

Be kind to yourself and concentrate on improvement rather than perfection.

In conclusion, setbacks are a normal part of any weight reduction journey, but it's easy to overcome them and maintain motivation with the correct mentality and tactics. To assist you in achieving your ultimate weight reduction objectives, celebrate your accomplishments, surround yourself with a supportive environment, control your triggers, and engage in self-compassion exercises.

Advice On Getting Over Ruts

A challenging aspect of any weight reduction journey is plateauing. When you put forth a lot of effort, eat well, and exercise often, you could discover that the scale eventually stops moving.

This happens often and may be demoralizing, but it's crucial to keep in mind that plateaus are a normal part of the process.

Our bodies are very adaptable, which is one of the major reasons plateaus happen. Our bodies adapt to the new calorie intake as we lose weight, and to preserve energy, our metabolism may slow down. This implies that to continue improving, we may need to change our eating habits and workout program.

There are many strategies you might use to break through a weight loss stall.

First and foremost, it's crucial to monitor your dietary consumption and activity schedule. This might assist you in determining any places where you would need to make changes. You may need to raise your exercise intensity or cut down on your calorie intake, for instance.

Changing up your workout program is another way to get beyond plateaus. Consider adding new exercises or upping the ante on your workout intensity. Your body may be shocked into burning more calories and breaking through the plateau if you do this.

It's critical to maintain your motivation throughout this period. While plateaus might be upsetting, it's important to keep in mind that they are a common aspect of the weight reduction process.

To remain on track, keep your attention on the progress you've already achieved and create modest, manageable objectives.

Lastly, it's critical to keep a pleasant attitude and a sound frame of mind. Keep in mind that losing weight is a journey and that setbacks are a normal part of the process. Be gentle to yourself and acknowledge your progress with modest successes.

You may overcome plateaus and succeed in your weight reduction objectives with perseverance and patience.

How To Remain Motivated When Losing Weight

It's typical to have ups and downs when trying to lose weight since it may be a difficult process. One of the greatest challenges individuals have is maintaining motivation when development seems to be stagnant.

While plateaus and setbacks are common throughout the weight reduction process, it's crucial to keep moving forward despite them.

It's crucial to establish reasonable objectives and recognize minor triumphs along the road if you want to remain motivated while losing weight.

Spend some time rewarding yourself for your efforts when you attain a goal. You may be motivated to keep going ahead as a result of this.

Finding a support system is a further useful method for maintaining motivation. Surround yourself with individuals who are supportive of your efforts to lose weight.

This may include close friends or relatives who are also trying to lose weight, a support group, or even a personal trainer. It might be quite beneficial to have someone to encourage you and keep you responsible.

Self-care and kindness toward oneself are also very essential. Avoid criticizing yourself for mistakes or failures. Instead, pay attention to your accomplishments and the distance you've come.

Spend some time unwinding, doing things you like, and placing a high priority on your mental and emotional wellness.

Last but not least, keep going even if you hit a wall or a setback. Instead, experiment with incorporating new activities into your regimen, switching up your diet, or consulting a healthcare provider for guidance.

Keep in mind that growth is not always linear and that it is OK to take a step back before continuing. You can overcome obstacles and maintain motivation on your weight reduction journey if you persevere and have a good outlook.

Using Failures As Fuel For Achievement By Learning From Them

Managing setbacks is one of the most difficult aspects of weight reduction. Along the road, challenges are inevitable, but it's crucial to keep in mind that your path need not be defined by setbacks.

In actuality, failures may provide a chance for learning, development, and a boost in motivation to accomplish your objectives.

Before anything else, it's critical to realize that setbacks are common and even anticipated throughout any weight reduction quest. Maybe you had a horrible day and ate too much junk food, or you were too busy and missed an exercise.

Whatever the setback may be, it's crucial to keep in mind that it's simply a single instance in time and doesn't represent your overall development.

It's crucial to stand back and reassess your objectives and tactics to overcome failures. Consider what may have contributed to the setback and how you might avoid it in the future.

Maybe you need to modify your diet or look for a new exercise regimen that better suits your interests and timetable.

With failures, it's also critical to maintaining positivity and motivation. Instead of punishing yourself for a mistake, try to concentrate on your development and the little triumphs you've already won.

Appreciate the wholesome decisions you've made and the beneficial adjustments to your body and mind.

Seeking assistance from others is another effective tactic for conquering obstacles. For support and inspiration, get in touch with a friend, a member of your family, or a support group.

The ability to remain on course and recover from failures depends greatly on having someone to share your journey with.

Finally, keep in mind that failures may be utilized as fuel for success. Make the most of your failures to develop and learn, and to strengthen your will to accomplish your objectives.

Each failure may help you learn something new about who you are and your path, and it can also make you stronger and more able to overcome obstacles.

In general, failures are an inevitable part of any weight reduction effort. You may overcome obstacles and go on your journey to a better and happier self by taking what you learned from them, keeping inspired, and getting help.

Conclusion: Points To Remember

We have covered a wide range of topics related to weight reduction in this book, including how to grasp the basic principles of weight loss, the function of calories, and metabolism. We also looked at how to make a sustainable diet plan and enjoy exercise.

We've also spoken about the value of having a positive outlook, establishing wholesome routines and habits, establishing a support network, dealing with setbacks, and maintaining motivation.

One of the main conclusions is that losing weight doesn't have to be challenging, but it does involve dedication to making lifestyle adjustments and creating a long-term strategy.

Setting attainable objectives, establishing wholesome routines and habits, coming up with a nutrition plan that suits your needs, choosing an activity you love, and establishing a support network are all part of this.

Another crucial idea is that shedding pounds involves more than just physical changes; it also involves mental and emotional well-being.

You may maintain motivation and concentration on your objectives by cultivating a positive outlook and learning to get through mental obstacles.

It's also important to keep in mind that obstacles come up naturally on any path, including the one to lose weight. Setbacks may be transformed into chances for development and advancement by learning from them and utilizing them as fuel for success.

Hence, to lose weight, one must adopt a comprehensive strategy that considers one's physical, mental, and emotional well-being.

You can successfully lose weight over the long term if you have a solid knowledge of the principles, establish healthy routines and habits, like exercising, maintain your motivation, and concentrate on your objectives.

Finally, Some Inspiring And Motivating Remarks.

I'm happy for you that you've started along the road to weight reduction. With that in mind, this is a marathon, not a race. Being patient with yourself is crucial, as is recognizing your progress's incremental successes.

Setbacks and plateaus are common throughout the process, so try not to let them demotivate you. Use the chance to get knowledge from them so that you may modify your method.

It's important to remember that losing weight involves not just physical changes, but also ones that affect one's thoughts and emotions. It's critical to maintain a good outlook, surround yourself with encouraging others, and concentrate on establishing long-lasting habits that will benefit you.

And last, constantly keep in mind that you can accomplish your objectives. Put your faith in the process and yourself. You've got this!